HOMEMADE SHAMPOOS

A Complete Organic Guide For Beginners

By

Linda Krall

INTRODUCTION

Making your own shampoos is not a new idea, in fact, it has been done by women and homemakers for thousands of years, before today's mass produced chemical based shampoos became available. A revival of interest in green living and healthy alternative products over the last few years has prompted a desire in many people to make their own shampoos and conditioners. The two biggest benefits of doing this is because of the huge savings that can be made by doing so and also to escape the horrific chemicals almost all commercial shampoos, conditioners and body products in general contain. The last chapter of this book details some of the harmful chemicals contained in many shampoos that should be avoided.

Shampoos come in many different types, made to suit all the different hair types from the beautify full black, curly wooly or frizzy hair common with many African Americans, the thick dark straight hair of many people of Asian descent and the light feathery hair with its many different shades of those people of European extraction. Hair comes in an array of textures, colors, lengths, and a multitude of variations, even from people within the same ethnic groups, as well as the newly form types from people with mixed and or different lineages. No particular ethnic group can claim to have better hair or have that their hair has any clear advantage over any other type, usually, but not always the hair and its color match the overall skin and body type of the person.

Some people tend to have naturally oily hair; others hair can be very dry. People's hair and skin color are passed down through the generations. The color and texture were first formed by the climatic conditions of the areas their ancestors originated from with people descending from the hotter areas of the planet tending to have darker skin color and hair darker and more curly or wavy hair. Nature has provided us with an internal sunscreen in the form of melanin, this group of compounds help to protect us from any harmful effects of the sun, the more melanin you have in your hair and skin the richer and darker your skin will be. Curly hair especially the tight very curvy types of hair allow for more airflow around the scalp providing a cooling effect.

It is a curious thing that many fair or white skinned people seek to actively darken their skin often through tanning and dying their hair as well as the use of cosmetics to make themselves feel and appear more attractive. Conversely many people with darker shades of skin avoid the sun and take measures to lighten their hair color and complexion.

Melanins are derivatives of the amino acid tyrosine; they are predominantly used in our bodies as protective pigments. Melanin's come in at least three naturally occurring types, eumelanin, pheomelanin, and neuromelanin, these determine the natural appearance, reflective quality, and color of an individual's hair, as well as affecting the hairs durability. Eumelanin is a dark pigment the most predominant melanins that are found in black and brunette hair (brown eumelanin and black eumelanin). When there is only a small amount of brown eumelanin and no other pigments it usually results in blond hair. Our hair can contain either eumelanin or pheomelanin, but not both, pheomelanin is a lighter pigment found in red hair, it can be found in concentrated amounts in the redder areas of the skin such as the lips. Because people with pheomelanin or red hair have less eumelanin pigment, their skin is generally quite pale and burns easily with sun exposure.

The range of colors produced by melanins is limited to shades of yellow, brown, red, and black, these when mixed together produce all the other natural hair colors.

Hair types are often broken into three main types, Asian, African and Caucasian hair types. Within these types, there are considerable variations such as the difference between the straight, thick hair common with Chinese and Japanese people to the thinner wavy hair common in people from Indonesia or the differences between Scandinavian hair types, which tend to be blond and the red hair common in Scotch people. Within the Melanesian population, it is quite common for people to have either very dark tightly curled hair, almost straight hair or even blond hair, often forming a natural "Afro Style". There are in fact people in all the different ethnic populations that have blond hair, red hair, straight hair and curly hair types, but these differences in the types of hair in each ethnic group are small compared to the main differences between Asian, African and Caucasian hair types. So hair types are usually classified into three main groups.

Asian hair tends to be less dense than the other types because the follicles are implanted causing the hair to grow straight, perpendicular to the scalp at an average speed of about 1.3cm per month making it the fastest growing type.

African people's hair tends to grow almost parallel to the scalp, often twisting around its self as it grows. It is a little denser on average than Asian hair and is the slowest growing type at about 0.9 cm per month.

European hair types grow at the rate of about 1.2 cm per month and are much denser that all other types. These follicles usually cause the hair to grow at an oblique angle to the scalp with a slight to moderately curve.

Specifically, the average density of afro-textured hair was found to be approximately 190 hairs per square centimeter. This was significantly lower than that of Caucasian hair, which, on average, has approximately 227 hairs per square centimeter

CONTENTS

CHAPTER 1

WASHING AND CARING FOR YOUR HAIR

How often you should wash your hair is a hotly debated question, there are many answers, depending on who you ask. The real answer is that it's not so simple, and there is not one answer, as everyone's hair is different, it really comes down to individual preferences and choices based on your own particular needs and the products you chose to use, your lifestyle and the environment you live and work in.

The fact is that the harsh chemicals used in many shampoos usually remove most the hair and more particularly the scalps natural oils and proteins in the process of cleaning, often causing the hair to dry out and become brittle and appear unhealthy. It then becomes necessary for these oils to be replaced, often with a chemical concoction that at best is a poor copy of the natural oils that were removed. Almost all the unnatural ingredients in commercially made shampoos and conditioners can over time prove to be a disadvantage when trying to maintain healthy hair and add additional toxins to our already polluted body's as a percentage of anything we put on our skin is absorbed into our system through our scalps, especially if warm or hot water is used.

Under normal circumstances, the longer you can leave your hair between washing the better, for those who work-out or come into contact with dust, grime or other contaminants it becomes necessary to clean the hair more often, so the mildest form of shampoo or cleaner possible should be used.

If you have thick curly hair, it can usually go without a wash for longer than fine, straight hair, other factors that can affect your hair are the amount of processing or artificial applications you have used on your hair. Coarse and curly or processed hair can restrict the easy movement of the natural oils produced by and present on your scalp, so they are not able to travel down the hair shaft as quickly as they could with fine straight hair. This often means that people feel the need to add extra oils to their hair to give it a healthy appearance

Personal comfort, hygiene, and appearances play a major role in when you decide to wash your hair, if you work-out daily or become sweaty, you will probably feel the need to wash your hair afterward. Those who have an oily scalp and thin, fine hair will often start to feel the need to wash their hair after about 24 hours to stop it looking flat and dirty, often it may be appropriate to use a dry cleaner instead of shampoo to clean the hair. Many people find that when they switch to a natural homemade shampoo, their scalp oil production will normalize. When the oils are stripped away each time the hair is washed, the scalp over produces new oils to compensate, with homemade shampoos it can take a few wash cycles to break this pattern, but soon they will find their natural level and the time between washing can be extended.

If you find your hair has become "frizzy" it is usually because the natural oils have been stripped out, when your scalp produces new oils which will help to tame these wild hair shafts over the next day or so your hair will start to improve and look better. Often people will apply hair gels or creams to calm their hair, when in reality just shampooing less frequently or using a milder shampoo would improve the look, feel and health of their hair and save on the need for using many other hair products.

People, who are lucky enough to have thick hair like most people of African descent have, will find that their scalp produces plenty of protective oils, called sebum. Studies have shown that African hair actually produces more oils than Caucasian and Asian types of hair. Very curly hair that can be found in all ethnic groups, often lacks the silky smoothness of straight hair, this is because, with tight curls, the natural oils are unable to spread evenly along the hair fibers and without adequate lubrication, the fibers can become very dry. This causes the brittle strands to flake and roughen, often resulting in hair that is coarse to the touch.

Hair thrives on oils and washing our hair too often results in us having to replenish the oils again. Using conventional methods, this can be very time consuming and expensive. A good solution is to use a dry cleaner and then to brush the hair gently so as not to damage the strands using a good quality brush. The old fashioned notion of brushing 100 strokes a day, provided it is done with care is an ideal way to distribute your own natural oils and remove any foreign objects.

The pH level (Potential of Hydrogen) of your hair and scalp oil sebum should be between 4.5 and 5.5 or acidic; studies have shown that an alkaline pH, anything above 7 which is considered "neutral," may increase the negative electrical charge of the hair fiber surface. This can increase friction between the fibers leading to cuticle damage and fiber breakage. Having a lower pH level in shampoos usually results in less friction between the hairs, the main cause of frizziness, this is particularly important for African hair and curly hair.

Inside the strand of each hair is a disulfide bond that determines the type and texture of your hair – straight, curly, fine or coarse hair – this natural disulfide bond is the cause of the appearance of people's hair. Disulfide bonds can be manipulated and changed by the use of chemicals such as those used to give perms or permanent changes such as chemical straighteners, and shampoos. These products must have the correct pH balance if the pH was very high it could cause the hair to simply disintegrate by destroying the disulfide bond.

Our bodies usually control dandruff or flaky, itchy, dry scalp, eczema, and psoriasis, these conditions are often caused by a fungus, if your sebum has a low pH level, but use a shampoo that has a pH that is too high the fungus will grow out of control, as fungus can't grow when there is a low pH it is best to, for this reason, to always use a shampoo or hair cleaning method that has a low or balanced pH level.

Although African hair is drier more brittle and susceptible to chemical and physical damage due to its spiral structure, it also has some advantages, especially in hot climates where it forms a natural barrier against the sun. Its shape, being a spiral curved form, has the effect of causing hot air to easily circulate through and around the scalp as part of the body's thermoregulatory mechanism, keeping the head cool. This hair shape also reduces the loss of fluids like water and sebum, so also helps with regulating the body's temperature.

Because of their gentle nature and healing capacity of all the shampoos in this book, they are ideal for use on hair that has been exposed to high amounts of heat through blow-drying or chemically treated hair, as well as dyed or bleached hair.

A good policy with most shampoos is to wash your hair using a small amount of shampoo and rinse it and then wash it again using more of the same shampoo. This is because the first wash stirs up skin cells, oil, and dirt, and the second wash cleans them away; then a conditioner can finish the job if needed.

CHAPTER 2

TYPES OF HOMEMADE SHAMPOOS AND RECIPES

Transition Period

Hair care is an individual and personal topic with everyone having their own unique body and hair makeup. When you first start changing from the commercial types of shampoos and conditioners with their heavy chemical components and high lather or foaming properties to a natural homemade type of shampoo, there is often a transition period that should be taken into account while your scalp and hair adjust.

Commercial products usually contain Sodium Laurel Sulfate, a chemically toxic surfactant or one of its derivatives, which are wetting and foaming agents. Their purpose is to allow the shampoo to spread out more easily and penetrate right into the hair; they also provide the lather or suds effect that many people now equate with cleaning power of efficiency; a fallacy created by manufacturing industry's to help them sell their products. Commercial shampoos are usually strong and harsh and have the action of just stripping the scalp and hair of all its vital oils, making it necessary to use a conditioner after shampooing in order to put these oils back into the hair to provide some level of "manageability". These conditioners used to correct the imbalance or lack of natural oils also usually contain more chemicals, creating a vicious cycle guaranteed to result in dry, brittle, lifeless hair and also possible damage to the skin, scalp and hair over time.

Because commercial shampoos have conditioned your scalp by removing all the natural oils every time you shampoo, causing the scalp to produce new sebum or the naturals oils to protect and nourish your hair, it often takes a few washes using new "green" or "chemical free" homemade shampoos before they "settle in" and begin to normalize or redevelop the natural cycles of scalp oil production. Sometimes it is necessary when you first begin using homemade shampoos to wash your hair every day to allow your scalp and hair to gradually adjust then slowly lengthening the days between washing until you building up to a wash cycle that is best for you.

With the gentle nature of these shampoos and the different needs of each individual, it may take a bit of trial and error until you find a shampoo that is easy for you to make and suits you and your individual hair type. Not all shampoos suit all hair types, but there is a natural homemade shampoo that is ideal for every hair type.

Coconut Milk Shampoos

Included are several recipes for coconut milk shampoo for those that wish to "go the whole way" as well as those that prefer to have a simpler version, but still get most of the benefits.

Coconut milk can be made from fresh coconuts, dried shredded coconut or even canned coconut milk, whichever type you use it is best to have an organic, unprocessed version for the best results

Unfortunately, castile soap and other soaps can react with certain minerals in some hard waters; this can form a film or residue and is the main reason apart from the price that most shampoo is made with "detergents," as detergents aren't as reactive to minerals in the water. The downside of using detergents is the harsh effect they can have and their other associated undesirable ingredients.

Coconut Milk and Castile Soap Shampoo

Ingredients

¼ of a cup of Coconut Milk

¼ of a cup of Castille Soap (Dr. Bronners is the most common)

20 drops of your favorite Essential Oil there are many that lend themselves to shampoos especially the different citrus and mints, lavender and rosemary

If you have dry hair, you can add a few drops of fresh organic oil such as olive, coconut, avocado, mango, almond or shea butter

Method

Combine all the ingredients in a food safe container and shake well until thoroughly combined. When using shake to remix and use approximately a tsp full each time you shampoo

Coconut Milk Shampoo

This shampoo recipe uses a readymade simple organic low pH shampoo (hopefully with the minimum amount of extra chemicals added), but transforms it into a very effective shampoo that is suitable for all hair types and can be used with "hard water."

Ingredients

¼ of a cup of coconut Milk

1/3 of a cup of mild Organic Shampoo

1 tsp of Olive, Palm or Almond Oil

10 to 290 drops of your favorite Essentials Oil

Method

Combine all the ingredients in a food safe container and shake well until thoroughly combined. When using shake to remix and use approximately a tsp full each time you shampoo

Coconut Milk and Aloe Vera Shampoo

An all-Natural pH Balanced Homemade Shampoo that is best made with fresh aloe vera pulp and fresh coconut milk, but if not available the canned variety can be used

Ingredients

¾ of a cup of Coconut Milk

¾ of a cup of Aloe Vera Pulp (Peel the fresh Aloe Vera and pulse for a few seconds in a blender to make a paste like consistency

15 to 20 drops of your favorite Essential Oil

Method

Wisk together in a bowl until totally combined and then pour it into ice cube trays and freeze it until solid. Once frozen place in an airtight container and use the free flow cubes of shampoo as required. It is best to remove them and thaw out before using.

After shampooing your hair, rinse it with a vinegar rinse using about 2 to 3 tbsp of vinegar to a liter of water. The recipe for making your own vinegar is at the start of the next chapter.

Hibiscus Shampoo

For thousands of years the people of Indonesia and India have used Hibiscus leaves and flowers to clean their hair, it is known to remove dirt without affecting the delicate balance of oils essential for the optimum health of your scalp and hair.

Ingredients

A large hand full of Hibiscus leaves (and a few flowers if you like)

Fresh clean, soft water

Method

Crush the Hibiscus leaves using your hands or if you like a paste and mortar. Then simmer the leaves in enough water to just cover them for about 20 minutes, allow it to cool strain it and massage it through your hair and onto your scalp, a nice lather will form, then rinse it away and repeat if desired.

Honey Shampoos

Honey shampoos are very simple to make and work exceptionally well, but should be made fresh as needed to avoid them spoiling. This is because honey will ferment when mixed with water. We always use Raw Unprocessed Honey, non-pasteurized, it should never be heated to a temperature hotter than you can comfortably put your hand in to avoid destroying the delicate enzymes in it that give it it's health related properties.

This "shampoo" is also exceptionally good as a lubricant when shaving delicate areas with a razor such as underarms, legs, and bikini lines.

Simple Honey Shampoo

Ingredients and method

Mix together 1 tbsp of raw honey with 3 tbsp of slightly warm, pure drinking water if you wish you can also add a few drops of your favorite Essential oil.

The mixture will be very watery and will not foam up, but this is how it is meant to be.

There is no need to use a conditioner, but if you like a rinse of Pineapple or apple cider vinegar can be used: see the recipe at the start of the next chapter.

Honey and Lemon Shampoo

Lemon juice is a natural hair moisturizer and conditioner; add 1 tbsp of fresh lemon juice or lemon juice concentrate and stir the mixture until completely combined; this will leave your hair healthy and shiny.

Honey and Rosewater Shampoo

Replace 1 or 2 tbsp of the water used to make the honey shampoo with Rosewater.

Liquid Potpourri Shampoo

Replace 1 or 2 tbsp of the water used to make the honey shampoo with liquid Potpourri and or add a tsp of Potpourri Oil to the shampoo and mix well to combine

Honey and Witch Hazel Shampoo

Make up a batch of Honey Shampoo, and add about a tsp of real Witch Hazel, it can be with just honey or combined with any of the other honey recipes to make you own unique shampoo.

Honey and Borax Shampoo

Any of the above shampoos can benefit with the addition of borax; it is best to dissolve 1 to 2 tsp of borax in warm (not hot) water before adding it to the honey.

Soap Nut Shampoo

Soap Nuts are not really a nut they are a close relative to the lychee a berry that grows on trees in the Himalayas because they contain saponin a naturally occurring cleaner that has many applications for those interested in a chemical free environment. Soapnuts are also known as Reetha Powder (Sapindus Mukorossi), the soap made from them is gentle on skin and hair without stripping the natural oils, making hair silky and shiny, without chemicals.

Ingredients and Method

Take two soapnuts and boil them in a cup of water for 15 minutes, then crush them or place them in a blender and puree them and then continue boiling for another 15 minutes.

Strain the liquid and reserve the leftover nuts, allowing them to dry out to be added to the next batch, they can be reused until they no longer release their born liquid.

The liquid left is a liquid soap, mix 4 tbsp into a cup of water to make Soapnut Shampoo.

This shampoo is so mild and yet effective it can be used as a whole body wash or to clean your clothes and dishes. Often Soapnut shampoo makes the hair look healthier and cleaner than any other shampoo.

Beer Shampoo

Beer shampoo is an old time remedy that was popular in the 50's; it was used for rejuvenating hair that had been dyed and permed using the harsh methods that were popular at that time. Today using beer in combination with some of the other homemade recipes in this book helps to add body and luster to hair. This shampoo will keep without refrigerating and may color light hair, so should be used on medium to dark hair colors where it can produce golden or tan highlights.

Ingredients

1 cup of Natural Beer of any type (leftover flat beer is fine for this recipe)

1 cup of Organic Natural Homemade Shampoo

Method

Reduce the beer by boiling in a saucepan until it's about ¼ of a cup.

Allow it to cool and add it to the shampoo mixing to combine.

Dried Herb Shampoo

This shampoo being organic in nature needs to be refrigerated once made, for average length hair use about 1 tbsp. the selection of herbs you choose is up to the individual. Some herbs are darker and may add to your hair color or bring new highlights to it.

For light colored hair it is recommended that light colored herbs such as Chamomile, Nettle or Lavender should be used, for darker hair Rosemary, Sage, Basil, etc. are suitable.

Ingredients and Method

Select about ½ a cup of your favorite dried herbs and pour a cup of boiling water over them, then allow them to sit and infuse for 30 minutes

Boil to sterilize 2 cups of fresh drinking water and then allow it to cool.

Strain the herb "tea" and place the liquid in a non-reactive bowl with the 2 cups of cooled water and ½ a cup of Castile Soap, grated Homemade Soap or Homemade Shampoo (if using grated soap it needs to soak until soft). Add 10 to 20 drops of your favorite Essential oil (optional) and for Dry Hair add 1 to 2 tsp of Coconut, Palm, Olive, Jojoba or Almond Oil. Then stir to completely combine before placing in a dispensing bottle.

Shake well before use

Egg Shampoo

This Shampoo helps add extra protein and body to your hair, wet your hair and gently rub the shampoo in with the tips of your fingers, then leave for 5 to 15 minutes and rinse out using warm water. It needs to be kept refrigerated and used within about 10 days so make a little at a time.

Ingredients

1 whole fresh Naturally Fed Organic Egg

1 tsp of cold pressed Olive, Palm or Coconut Oil

1 tbsp of Homemade Shampoo or a mild Organic Green unscented Commercial Shampoo

½ a cup of Fresh Drinking Water

Method

Place all the ingredients in a blender or use a blending stick to blend into a smooth liquid

Jojoba Oil Shampoo (for dry Hair)

Jojoba Oil shampoo is made for dry hair; it helps to moisturize and condition the hair and provides an additional body for hair that has been damaged by heat and chemical treatments. I will not lather up in the same way as commercial shampoo and should be kept in a food safe airtight container.

Ingredients

2 tbsp of Homemade or Mild Unscented Organic Shampoo

1 tsp of Jojoba Oil

1 tsp of Coconut Oil

1 tsp of Glycerin

½ of a cup of Distilled or Filtered Drinking Water

Method

Place all the ingredients in a bowl and stir them to mix thoroughly and place in an airtight food safe container.

Witch Hazel and Indian Herb Shampoo

The herbs that are used in this shampoo were selected because of their well-known properties of helping to cleanse, moisturize, repair and volumize hair in a natural, healthy manner. This is volume type shampoo that is best used on dry hair, so do not wet your hair first, just pour about half a cup of the shampoo on your dry hair and gently massage it through from scalp to the tips of the hair, but concentrate mainly on our scalp. It is suggested that you then rinse your hair well and lightly towel dry it and then apply a second amount sufficient to saturate the hair and scalp. This should also be gently massaged into your hair, but concentrating on your scalp. Rinse thoroughly and gently dry the hair.

Ingredients

1 tbsp of ground Shikakai Pods (Shikakai means "fruit of the hair")

1 tbsp of ground Reetha (soapnut)

¾ of a tbsp of Amla, (Indian Gooseberry)

½ a tbsp of Neem Powder (this is used because it helps to reduce scalp itchiness, enhances the growth of the hair and also helps to prevent dandruff and lice)

¼ of a tsp of Ceylon Cinnamon (has anti-fungal and antibacterial properties to benefit the scalp and combat hair loss).

Bouquet Garni made of 2 Bay leaves, 2 Basil Leaves and 2 Sprigs of fresh Rosemary

5 to 8 drops of your favorite Essential Oils

3 cups plus 2 cups of fresh filtered drinking water

Method

Place 2 cups of water in a medium-sized saucepan and add the herbs then bring to a very slow simmer. The mixture will foam a little but try to avoid it boiling over. Allow this to simmer for about 15 minutes and then strain it out into a large bowl through a colander lined with cheesecloth or a wet tea towel. You should end up with about a cupful of shampoo. Allow it to cool to a temperature you can place your finger in and then add the Essential oils and the additional cups of water. Your shampoo is now ready to use.

The ultimate Bar Soap Shampoo

This bar soap shampoo has been developed to cater for the whole family it is excellent as a men's, women's and children's shampoo. It has excellent properties making it ideal for washing beards and facial hair. This shampoo is ideally suited to be used in conjunction with finishing rinses such as an apple cider vinegar or lemon juice rinse.

Extreme Caution Needs to be used when making soaps especially those that contain Lye or Caustic Soda it is potentially very dangerous and can cause serious burns loss of eyesight and intense pain.

USE PROTECTIVE OR SAFTY GEAR INCLUDING GLOVES AND SAFTY GLASSES AND TAKE EXTREME CAUTION. <u>CAREFULLY ADD THE LYE INTO THE OTHER LIQUID AND GENTLY STIR TO COMBINE. DO NOT ADD THE LIQUID TO THE LYE IT CAN REACT BADLY CAUSING IT TO ERUPT AND CAUSE SERIOUS BURNS.</u>

Note the reaction that occurs will cause the mixture to get very hot so the container or bowl will also be hot. THIS LIQUID IS CAUSTIC AND **SHOULD NOT BE ALLOWED TO COME INTO CONTACT WITH THE SKIN AND THE FUMES SHOULD NOT BE INHALED.**

Have some vinegar on hand in case of spills as vinegar will neutralize the lye

Ingredients (by Weight)

9 oz of cold-pressed Coconut Oil

9 oz of cold pressed Virgin Olive Oil

5 oz of Castor Oil

3 oz of Jojoba Oil

2 oz of Shea Butter

2 oz of Cocoa Butter

1 oz of Bees Wax

4 oz of Filtered Drinking Water or Herb water

6 oz of Coconut Milk or Goats Milk

4 oz of Lye (Caustic Soda)

Optional Essential Oils

Any of you favorite Essential can be used but as a guide, it is recommended that you use these or similar

For blond hair use Lemon and Lavender

For dark hair use Rosemary and Peppermint

For all hair types use Lime and Coconut

Method

Combine the water and coconut milk in a large non-reactive bowl (glass is best)

Using extreme caution, Measure out by weight place the lye into a glass measuring cup

Very carefully and slowly in a well-ventilated area (preferably outside) add the lye to the liquid and gently stir it to combine, do not touch the liquid in any way.

Measure out all of the Oils by weight (it is best to use kitchen scales and also use the same scales of everything in this recipe).

The oils should be combined with the beeswax in a saucepan and then placed on a very low heat until they are completely melted and stirred to combine. They should then be poured into a crockpot (slow electrical cooker) that is set to its lowest setting but do not allow them to get too hot.

Very slowly using extreme care pour the liquid and lye mixture into the oils in the crockpot and stir then gently to combine. Once they are totally combined, they can be blended using a stick blender. They need to be blended until they start to thicken and form a trace. This means that when the mixture is stirred, there is a pattern or wake left so you can clearly see where you have stirred. Another way of telling if it is ready is to take a spoonful of the mixture and pouring it back onto the surface of the mixture. If it stays on the surface like a drop of water would on a piece of glass it is ready. The soap will now have the consistency of a thick pudding.

Place the lid on the crockpot and cook the soap on the lowest setting for an hour.

At the end of the cooking time, the soap will look completely transparent. When this happens, turn off the crockpot and prepare the molds. If you do not have molds any small heatproof containers can be used, first give them a generous coat of coconut oil.

Before you pour the molds add any essential oils you would like in the soap, it is quite possible to divide the soap and use different essential oils in each mold giving the finished products different distinct perfumes.

Spoon the soap into the molds and allow them to harden or set for at least 24 hours at which time you can cut the soap into whatever shape you desire.

The soap should be stacked so it can get a good airflow to further cure, but you can now test the soap. It should be mild, but if you find it has a bit of tang it means it needs to cure further.

Coconut and Olive Oil Soap

This soap is an excellent homemade soap to use as a base for your homemade shampoos

Ingredients

9 ounces of coconut oil

21 ounces of olive oil

9 ounces of clean, fresh drinking water

4.1 ounces of sodium hydroxide, also called lye

Fragrance; your choice of Essential oils (optional)

A soap mold or container for the soap to set in (optional)

Method

It is a good idea to have your mold or molds ready before you start mixing the soap as it can solidify very quickly once mixed.

Heat the oils to 43C (110F), or until they are completely fluid.

Mix the Lye, using your safety gear (rubber gloves and eye protection), place the water in your non-reactive bowl and slowly mix in the sodium hydroxide, or lye, this will help to prevent splashing and burns. This mixture will heat up by itself. When it is thoroughly mixed, allow it to cool to 43C (110F).

With the oils and lye mixture are both at 43C (110F), slowly add the oils to the lye, and use a stick or immersion blender to mix them together until they do not separate about 3 minutes. This can be done with a whisk or hand beater, but this takes much longer. When there is a trace (when the soap mixture is stirred a visible line is left in the mixture or when a drop of the mixture is taken and gently place back on the surface and does not sink back in, but sits on the surface, like a drip of honey placed on a plate), and no streaks of oil are left in the mixture. It is ready to pour into the mold or molds.

Pour the mixture into the mold quickly, and then wrap them in a towel to set for 24 hours. After the soap has set, it can be cut into the shapes you desire. At this stage, the soap is still caustic, so it is best to put on your gloves to protect your hands. The best method I have found to cut the soap is a steal guitar string tied between two sticks; this will easily slice the soap. After cutting, or if you used sized molds, allow the soaps to dry for between 3 and 4 weeks, to balance the pH level of the soap making it safe for use.

CHAPTER 3

NATURAL HOMEMADE CONDITIONERS

Hair conditioners are necessary for most commercial shampoos and many shampoos now include conditioners in with the shampoo. Most homemade shampoos because they do not destroy or remove the natural oils do not need to be followed by a conditioner, some benefit from the use of a vinegar or citrus based rinse to restore the natural pH levels which for most people are between 4.5 and 6, with 7 being neutral and over that is acidic which allows fungus molds and pests to survive.

Vinegar is an ideal natural conditioner and is best used in a diluted form of about 1 to 3 tablespoons to a liter of water; the softer the water (lower the mineral content), the less vinegar is needed. Another very good basic conditioner is lemon or other citrus juices. All types of vinegar can be used; however below are two very easy vinegars that can be made at home using scraps that would otherwise be discarded into the trash.

Apple Cider Vinegar

Apple cider vinegar is so easy to make, it can be made from any part of an apple from the whole apple or just the skins, but care should be used in choosing the apples you use, because they are on the list of the most toxin-laden foods, so Certified Organic apples or better yet apples from your own or friends trees should be used. During the seasons when apples are cheap and plentiful, it is the best time to make vinegar as once made it will keep indefinitely and has many uses around an organic home. By using the skins, cores and other parts that are usually not eaten you can really get your vinegar for free. Often apples that are overripe can be purchased from store or markets for almost nothing. If you only have a few skins and cores they can be frozen until you have collected enough to make a batch of vinegar.

Ingredients

The skins and cores from enough Apples to 3/4 fill the jar or food safe container you have.

Fresh Pure Water

Method

Place all the apple you wish to use, skins, trimmings and cores in a bowl, and let them sit in the air until they turn brown, covered with a piece of cheesecloth to keep insects away.

When they have turned brown a day or so place them into a clean jar or food safe container and cover them with fresh, clean water. Then cover the bowl with cheesecloth or fine linen and secure it with a rubber band or twine. Leave the jar for about 4 to 6 weeks to ferment in a warm dark place.

After about 4 weeks the vinegar will be ready for a taste test. Taste it and decide if it's strong enough, or you want to leave it a while longer. When the vinegar is at a strength you like, strain it through cheesecloth or fine linen and discard the solids. Often the vinegar will be cloudy, this is normal, as it has the "Mother Culture" living in it, it will settle to the bottom in a few days, but if you want the vinegar clear, strain it through a coffee filter. It is a good idea to keep the "Mother" in a little of the vinegar as a starter for your next vinegar.

Bottle the vinegar in clean jars or food safe containers. First, wash the containers with bicarbonate soda and then rinse them thoroughly, this removes any soap or other residues then sterilize them; a pressure cooker is ideal for sterilizing them. Once bottled, keep the vinegar in a cool darkish place where it will keep indefinitely.

Pineapple Vinegar

Ingredients

1 & 1/2 liters of Pure Fresh Water

3/4 of a Cup of Organic Raw Sugar

The peel and trimmings of 1 Whole Organic Pineapple

1 2 lit plus Jar or food safe container to make the Vinegar in

Method

The rough skin of pineapple means they need to be washed, the best method is by scrubbing the pineapple with a stiff brush to remove any dirt or mold using a solution of 1 tbsp of thyme and 1 tbsp of vinegar per liter of water, (no soap or detergent).

Wash the jars or food safe containers you wish to store the vinegar in with bicarbonate soda, and then rinse them in clean in fresh water. Dissolve the sugar in the water and place this in the jar or jars you will use. Place all scraps from your pineapple, skin, eyes, core and other trimmings in the jar, and stir or shake it to mix well. Place a piece of cheesecloth, or similar over the top of the jar and secure it with a rubber band or twine, to keep insects out. Then allow it to sit undisturbed it in a warm darkish place for 2 to 6 weeks, depending on the outside temperature. During this time the mixture may turn murky and brownish, this is quite normal it is only the "Mother Culture", do not shake the jar.

When the liquid clears or after 3 weeks, do a taste test and decide if you are happy with the strength and flavor of your vinegar. Decide if you wish to slow down the process, then or allow it to continue, the vinegar will become stronger the longer you leave it, to slow the process pour the vinegar through several layers of cheesecloth removing all solids and store in a clean bottle out of direct sunlight.

The Mother or white mass that floats on the surface or lies on the bottom is harmless. It is the culture that produces the vinegar, it is a good idea to save this for your next batch of vinegar as a starter, and this will shorten the time it takes for the brew to be made.

Mayonnaise, Egg whites, and Yogurt Conditioner

This conditioner is best made with homemade or organic mayonnaise and yogurt, but if desired different flavored yogurt can be used. The conditioner is of a runny or sloppy consistency, so it requires a shower cap or a damp towel to cover your head to keep it in place for the 30 minutes plus that is needed for it to perform its magic. It is important to also rinse and a final rinse in warm water, not in hot water.

Ingredients

½ a cup of Yogurt, standard Organic or Coconut Milk Yogurt

½ a cup of Homemade or Organic Mayonnaise

1 large Organic Egg white

Method

Place all the ingredients in a bowl and or your blender and blend or whip them until they become smooth.

Wash your hair with your chosen shampoo and gently dry your hair, then massage the conditioner into your hair it is best to try and coat all the hair strands and massage into the scalp. Place on a shower cap or a large wet towel to keep the conditioner in place. Then after 30 minutes start to rinse the conditioner off with warm NOT HOT water, it may need several rinses.

Coconut Oil Conditioner for Oily Hair

Coconut oil is one of the few vegetable oils that is good for hair; it will make it shiny and soft as well as giving some protection from parasites. This coconut conditioner is especially good at getting rid of excess oil and leaving your hair looking and feeling fresh light and natural.

Ingredients

1 Free Range Organic Egg Yolk

1 tsp of cold pressed Coconut Oil

1 cup of fresh filtered Drinking Water

Method

Whisk the egg yolk until frothy and then whisk in the oil and water until it becomes smooth. Wash your hair with the shampoo of your choice and gently dry it, then massage the conditioner through you hair and scalp. Allow it to rest for 3 to 6 minutes and rinse it out in cool water.

Avocado Conditioner

Avocados are not only great to eat, but they also give your hair the benefit of their healthy oils, transforming dull, difficult hair into shiny, manageable healthy soft hair.

Ingredients

1 ripe Avocado

2 tbsp of cold pressed Olive or Coconut Oil

2 tbsp of fresh whole fat full Organic Cream

2 tbsp of fresh filtered Drinking Water

Method

Place all the ingredients in a small bowl and whisk them together and massage it into your hair and cover it with a damp towel, allow it to penetrate into your hair and follicles for about

20 to 30 minutes then rinse the conditioner out with warm (Not Hot) water.

Baking Soda Shampoo

Baking soda is one of the simplest most affordable and effective nontoxic shampoos available; it leaves your hair clean and fresh if followed by a vinegar rinse it is a great solution for people who do not want all the chemicals in most commercial shampoos. It is very good for removing any buildup or residues from other shampoos. A few people suggest that it may cause itchy scalp because it tends to dry out the skin and it is not suitable for everyday washing but very effective once a week.

Ingredients and method

Mix 1 tbsp of baking soda with 1 cup of warm water and massage it into your scalp and hair. If you wish to make a large amount mix ½ a cup of baking soda with 3 cups of water.

Borax shampoo

This is a very effective shampoo and works very well if you massage a small amount of coconut oil into your hair, place a little in a finger bowl and dip the tips of your fingers in the oil and massage it through your hair and then leave it for a few hours or overnight. Then wet the hair with cool or warm water and place a damp hand into a bowl of dry borax, you will get a good coating stuck to your hand and just rub this into your damp hair. It will very quickly lather up because of the reaction between the coconut oil and the borax giving a very soft lather it will leave your hair soft and manageable.

Citrus Shampoo and all-purpose Wash

From whenever the fresh citrus fruit is available, we make our own lemonade, orangeade, of whatever "citrus-ade" each week, but after making the juice instead of throwing away the pith peel and other bits we cannot eat, we make our citrus shampoo and all-purpose cleaner.

To make the shampoo / cleaner, first simmer the skins and any other parts you do not eat, in water for about 4 hours, and then allow them to cool and stand or leave them overnight. This makes fruit water, which is full of natural oils and fruit acids. Once you have made your fruit water, strain it to remove all the solids, and then place a cup full of it in a high sided bowl (as it will foam up a bit), and then slowly add about 1 & 1/2 to 2 cups of baking soda to it to form a smooth paste.

This shampoo is basically citric acid, a very effective cleaner; you only need a very small amount to cut through the dirt and grime in your hair. Then rinse thoroughly and apply a small amount of coconut, palm or olive oil. If preferred a few drops of your favorite essential oil can be added provide an individual or a different smell.

Natural dry Shampoo

This natural dry shampoo is pH balanced to help keep your hair fresh and clean between wet washes.

Ingredients

2 tsp of organic Corn Starch

2 tbsp of organic Rice Flour

2 tbsp of organic Arrowroot Powder

1 tbsp of Baking Soda

8 to 12 drops of your favorite Essential Oil

For Dark hair add 2 tbsp of Cocoa Powder

Method

Combine all the ingredients making sure the essential oil in well incorporated without any lumps. When you apply the dry powder shampoo be sure the scalp and hair are completely dry, sprinkle a little onto the scalp and gently massage it into the hair and scalp area. Once the whole scalp and all the hair has been covered with the powder, using a medium to stiff brush, brush out the powder along with any dirt and impurities on your scalp or in your hair.

CHAPTER 4

NATURAL SHAMPOO ADDITIONS

To control Oily Hair, use 2 organic egg yolks mixed with 2 tsp of fresh lemon juice or organic raw vinegar and gently work it into the hair, allow it to work for a few minutes then wash it out using a warm (Not Hot) shower.

If you find you have excessive oil in the hair wet the hair and sprinkle borax powder liberally through the hair and rub it into a lather and rinse with warm (Not Hot) water,

The addition of 8 to 12 drops of citrus essential oils to your shampoo will help it to remove excess oil from your hair without stimulating the production of more oil.

When using homemade shampoos, it is necessary to shake or stir them each time you use them as they are free from the chemicals that bind the shampoo together so are likely to split back to their raw forms. A simple remixing will restore all shampoos to original condition.

If you find your homemade shampoo it too thin and would like to thicken it up

You can blend a small amount of whole oats in a good blender and then mix in a small amount of baking soda and water. Slowly add this mixture to your shampoo until you reach your desired thickness.

Cornstarch or arrowroot powder mixed with the baking soda and water can also be added a little at a time to thicken shampoos and or conditioners.

CHAPTER 5

TOXIC CHEMICALS FOUND IN SHAMPOOS

Nowadays it is very important to check the labels as almost all soaps and shampoos contain a variety of toxic chemicals, artificial scents, and colorings. A large proportion, about 90% of all shampoos and of soaps contain a detergent called sodium lauryl sulfate or SLS this nasty chemical is absorbed by the skin; it penetrates into the eyes, brain, heart, and liver. It has been positively linked to causing cataracts, eye damage, and cancers. SLS does not have to enter the eye directly as it is able to be readily absorbed by the skin. SLS is the main ingredient in most baby shampoos. This dangerous chemical enhances the absorption of all other chemicals into your body. Many body products contain another additive, Propylene Glycol; this is often in baby wipes, lotions, and many cosmetic products. Propylene Glycol is known to cause skin rashes, deafness, kidney damage and liver problems, this chemical damages cell membranes which is of special concern.

Other Nasties in many "body care" products

Methylisothiazolinone – Is an environmental toxin which irritates the skin, eyes, and lungs as well as causing brain damage.

Methylchloroisothiazolinone – Is carcinogenic as well as an environmental toxin and allergen/Irritant.

Cocamide Mea – Is carcinogenic, it damages the reproductive system and organ systems.

CocamidopropylBetaine - CocamidopropylDimethylamine – Is an environmental and immune system toxin as well as being an allergen.

3-Dimethylamino-propylamine – Is an immune system and Organ toxin, an allergen and irritates the skin, eyes, and lungs.

Nitrosamines – Is carcinogenic, it damages the reproductive and organ systems.

Ammonium Laureth Sulfate – Sodium Laureth Sulfate.

Ethylene Oxide – Is carcinogenic, A reproductive, immune and respiratory system toxin/irritant.

1,4-Dioxane – Is carcinogenic, an allergen, immune, and organ system toxin

D&C Red 33–Coal Tar dye – It causes asthma and is a known carcinogenic.

Dimethicone – Is an environmental and organ system toxin.

TetrasidiumEdta – Enhances the absorption of all other chemicals and is an organ system toxin.

Sodium Benzoate – Is an organ system toxin.

Blue 1 – FD&C Blue No1 –There are toxicity reports by the FDA and it causes deaths.

Sodium Xylene Sulfonate – Is a lung and skin irritant, it also causes liver toxicity.

Polyquaternium 76 – May contain harmful impurities or form toxic breakdown products linked to cancer or other significant health problems. Found in body products.

Glycol Distearate – Environmental toxin, very limited information available???

Zea Mays Corn Extract – If it is organic, that is OK, but GM forms have high concentrations of Glyphosate

Hydrolyzed Silk – There are no known reports or information about toxicity.

CONCLUSION

Shampoos are not only expensive but full of all different combinations of nasty chemicals. Our family has not used any store bought shampoos or conditioners for several years. After going through many different brands of natural commercial shampoos and conditioners and finding that all of those tend to be quite pricey, we have settled on using most of the shampoos in this book as our family has a variety of hair types.

Having school-age children means hair care is on a whole new level. No matter how clean their hair is, they come home from school with a number of different things in their hair. Itchy scalp, dandruff, head lice, paint, glue and general grime. I have developed a washing routine that keeps their hair clean and fresh based on the recipes in this book. Apart from the health aspects, we have enjoyed the substantial savings we can see by no longer purchasing soaps, shampoos, and conditioners from the supermarket or specialty stores. These shampoos are so easy and inexpensive to make that it is worth it to put the time and effort into making them and knowing what ingredients are in the bottle. As most of the ingredients are things that are easily available and probably already in your home, you will also see a difference in your grocery bill when you no longer have to purchase these with your weekly shopping list.

I would like to thank you for reading it and hope you found some enjoyment and useful information to help with your new regimen in hair management.